MW01420818

Nutrition and Weight Management Journal

Mayfield Publishing Company
Mountain View, California
London • Toronto

International Standard Book Number 0-7674-0743-1

Manufactured in the United States of America
10 9 8 7 6 5 4 3 2

Mayfield Publishing Company
1280 Villa Street
Mountain View, California 94041
(650) 960-3222

Contents

HOW TO USE THIS JOURNAL

Nutrition is a vitally important component of wellness. Diet influences energy levels, well-being, and overall health. A well-planned diet supports maximum fitness and protects against disease. The first part of this journal is designed to help you analyze your current eating habits, to identify patterns that may be causing you to shortchange yourself on nutrition, and to put a more balanced eating plan into action.

The second part of this journal covers *weight management.* You may have a goal for your weight that is above or below your current weight. You can develop a plan to manage your weight and keep a weight management log in the second part of this journal. You will find the information you gathered in keeping your nutrition logs helpful in completing a weight management plan.

To start monitoring, assessing, and improving your nutritional habits, follow these steps:

1. Review the tools for keeping a nutrition log contained in the first section of this booklet.
2. Using this information, fill out the Preprogram Nutrition Log by tracking your diet for 3 days.
3. Use the Assessing Your Daily Diet worksheets to analyze your daily nutritional intake. Do you see some areas in your current diet that could be improved?
4. Complete the Behavior Change Contract, using the Tools for Improving Your Food Choices section to identify unhealthy behaviors and to plan how to improve them.
5. Record your daily diet a second time.
6. Analyze your revised diet and compare it to your original diet.

Once you understand your nutritional needs and habits, you can make reasonable and healthy choices for weight management.

NUTRITION

TOOLS FOR MONITORING YOUR DAILY DIET

The Food Guide Pyramid

Use the Food Guide Pyramid as a guide to daily food choices. The Pyramid is an outline of what to eat each day—not a rigid prescription, but a general guide that lets you choose a healthful diet that's right for you. It calls for eating a variety of foods to get the nutrients you need and at the same time the right amount of calories to maintain a healthy weight.

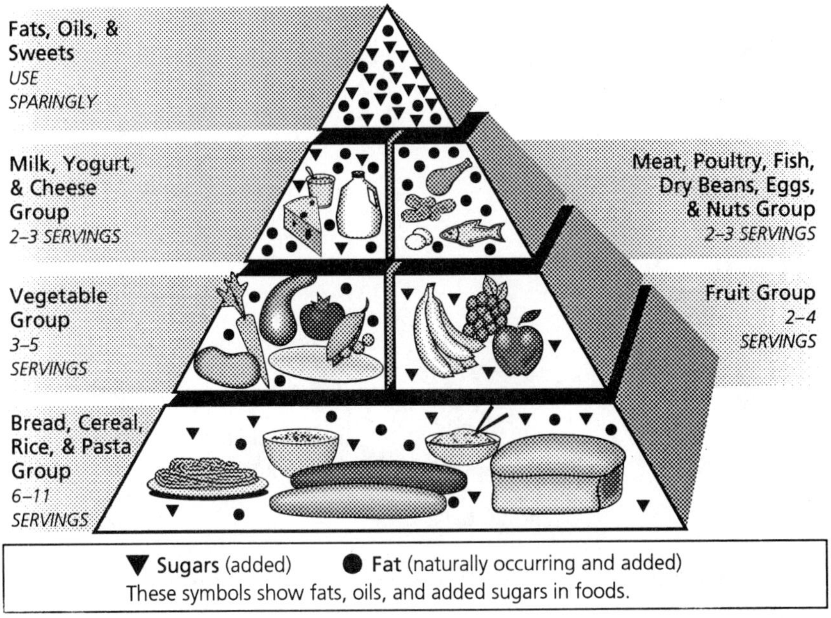

Food Groups and Recommended Servings

The recommendations of the Pyramid are based on serving sizes. Refer to this table for the recommended number of servings and some examples of serving sizes for each group:

Food Group	Number of Servings	Foods and Serving Sizes
Milk, yogurt, and cheese	2–3	1 cup milk 1 1/2 oz cheese 2 oz processed cheese 1 cup yogurt
Meat, poultry, fish, dry beans, eggs, and nuts	2–3*	2–3 oz cooked meat, poultry, fish 1–1 1/2 cups cooked dry beans 4 tbsp peanut butter 2 eggs 1/2–1 cup nuts
Fruits	2–4	1 whole piece of fruit 1 melon wedge 1/2 cup berries 1/2 grapefruit 1/4 cup dried fruit 1/2 cup cooked or canned fruit 3/4 cup juice
Vegetables	3–5	1/2 cup raw or cooked vegetables 1 cup raw leafy vegetables 3/4 cup juice
Bread, cereals, rice, and pasta	6–11	1 slice of bread 1/2 hamburger bun, English muffin, or bagel (depending on size) 1 small roll, biscuit, or muffin 1 oz ready-to-eat cereal 1/2–3/4 cup cooked cereal, rice, or pasta 3–4 small or 2 large crackers
Fats, oils, and sweets	Foods from this group should not replace any from the other groups. Amounts consumed should be determined by individual energy needs.	

*Your total daily intake should be the equivalent of 5–7 ounces of cooked lean meat, poultry, or fish. The following portions of nonmeat foods are equivalent to 1 ounce of lean meat: 1 egg, 2 tbsp peanut butter, 1/3 cup nuts, 1/4 cup seeds, 1/2 cup tofu.

When you use the table on the previous page to determine the number of servings you should be eating from each food group, remember that the range of servings is designed to accommodate a range of calorie levels depending on age, gender, and level of activity. The low end of the recommended range of servings is about right for many sedentary women and older adults; the middle of the range is about right for most children, teenage girls, active women, and many sedentary men; and the top of the range is about right for teenage boys, many active men, and some very active women.

Making Choices Within the Food Groups

As shown in the Food Groups and Recommended Servings table, you can choose from a variety of foods in each food group to fulfill your daily needs. The average American diet is at or below the low end of the servings range for most food groups, but we eat too much fat and added sugars to meet the recommendations without gaining weight. The key is to make better food choices within the groups and so get more nutrients for your calories. Keep these guidelines in mind as you plan your meals:

General

- Choose a variety of foods within each group. Different foods contain different combinations of nutrients.
- If you are concerned about eating too much and gaining weight, concentrate on nutrient-dense foods—foods that are high in nutrients relative to the amount of calories they contain.

Milk, yogurt, and cheese

- Pick skim milk and nonfat yogurt over whole milk and regular yogurt.
- Choose "part skim" or low-fat cheeses, ice milk, and frozen yogurt over their higher-fat counterparts.

- If calcium intake is a concern, remember that cottage cheese is lower in calcium than many other dairy products.

Meat, poultry, fish, dry beans, eggs, and nuts

- The choices lowest in fat in this group are lean meat, skinless poultry, fish, and dry beans and peas.
- Trim the fat from meat and prepare it by broiling, roasting, or boiling.
- Use egg yolks, nuts, and seeds in moderation.

Fruits

- Choose fresh fruits, fruit juices, and frozen, canned, or dried fruit over fruit in heavy syrups or sweetened fruit drinks.
- For a higher fiber intake, choose whole fruits over fruit juices often.
- Choose citrus fruit, melons, and berries for vitamin C.

Vegetables

- To take advantage of the different nutrients found in different types of vegetables, include servings of each type in your diet regularly: dark-green leafy vegetables, deep-yellow vegetables, starchy vegetables, legumes, and other vegetables.
- Choose dark-green leafy vegetables and legumes often; they are especially rich in vitamins and minerals.

Bread, cereals, rice, and pasta

- For a healthy fiber intake, choose several servings a day of foods made from whole grains.
- Choose most often foods with little fat or sugar, such as bread, rice, and pasta.

- Limit your consumption of baked goods included in this group but high in fat and sugar such as cakes, cookies, croissants, and pastries.
- Try preparing packaged pasta, stuffing, and sauces using half the butter suggested or low-fat milk in place of milk or cream.

Self-Assessment: Portion Size Quiz

Now test yourself to see if your perception of serving sizes is the same as those used with the Food Guide Pyramid (check your answers on the next page). Remember that when you keep your nutrition log you will need to assess your intake using the Pyramid serving sizes.

1. An ounce and a half of hard cheese—equivalent to one serving from the dairy group—looks most like
   a. one domino.
   b. two dominoes.
   c. three dominoes.
2. A half cup of cooked pasta, considered a serving from the grain group, most easily fits into
   a. an ice cream scoop (the kind with a release handle).
   b. a ball the size of a medium grapefruit.
   c. a cereal bowl.
3. One drink of wine roughly fills
   a. two-thirds of a coffee cup.
   b. one coffee cup.
   c. two coffee cups.
4. One serving of green grapes consists of how many grapes?
   a. 10
   b. 15
   c. 20

5. Three ounces of beef, a serving's worth, most closely resembles
   a. a *T.V. Guide.*
   b. a regular bar of soap.
   c. a small bar of soap (as from a hotel).
6. One serving of brussels sprouts consists of how many sprouts?
   a. 4
   b. 8
   c. 12
7. Two tablespoons of olive oil more or less fill
   a. a shot glass.
   b. a thimble.
   c. a Dixie cup.
8. Two tablespoons of peanut butter make a ball the size of
   a. a marble.
   b. a tennis ball.
   c. a Ping-Pong ball.
9. How many shakes of a five-hole salt shaker does it take to reach 1 teaspoon (approximately the maximum amount of salt recommended per day)?
   a. 5
   b. 10
   c. 60
10. There are eight servings in a loaf of Entenmann's Raspberry Danish Twist. A serving is the width of
   a. one finger.
   b. two fingers.
   c. four fingers.

Answers

1. c	3. a	5. b	7. a	9. c
2. a	4. b	6. a	8. c	10. b

Food Labels

Another important tool for keeping your nutrition log is the information you will find on food labels. In the example below, note that the serving size is 1/2 cup. If you eat 2 cups of macaroni and cheese, you'll need to record that you ate a total of 4 servings. Other useful information includes total calories and calories from fat per serving. Remember that the serving size given on the food label is often not the same as the serving size specified by the Food Guide Pyramid, and neither one may be the size of the serving you choose for yourself.

Standardized serving size.

Calories from fat shows how much fat the food contains.

% Daily Value indicates how much of a day's worth of the listed items the food provides in terms of a daily diet of 2,000 calories. A guide for evaluating daily intake for these items is shown in the table below.

Nutritional values for these items enable consumers to evaluate the food for "good" and "bad" nutrient content.

This table shows recommended daily intake for two levels of calorie consumption. It's the same on all labels.

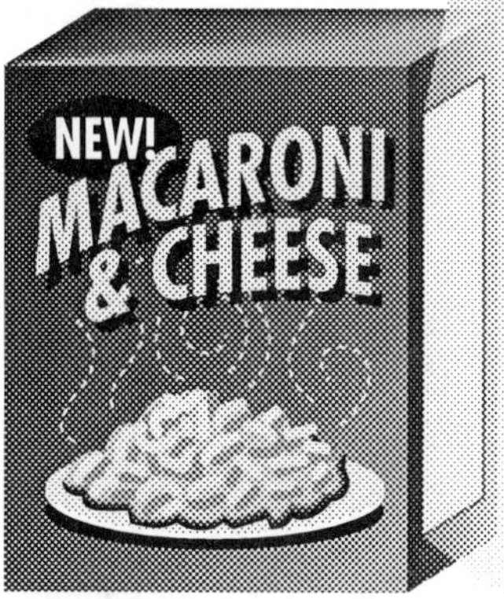

Numbers for dietary calculations.

Nutrition Facts

Serving Size 1/2 cup (114g)
Servings per Container 4

Amount per Serving

Calories 260 Calories from Fat 120

	% Daily Value*
Total Fat 13g	**20%**
Saturated Fat 5g	**25%**
Cholesterol 30mg	**10%**
Sodium 660mg	**28%**
Total Carbohydrate 31g	**11%**
Sugars 5g	
Dietary Fiber 0g	**0%**
Protein 5g	

Vitamin A 4% • Vitamin C 2% • Calcium 15% • Iron 4%

*Percents (%) of a Daily Value are based on a 2,000 calorie diet. Your Daily Values may vary higher or lower depending on your calorie needs:

Nutrients		2,000 Calories	2,500 Calories
Total Fat	Less than	65g	80g
Sat Fat	Less than	20g	25g
Cholesterol	Less than	300mg	300mg
Sodium	Less than	2,400mg	2,400mg
Total Carbohydrate		300g	375g
Fiber		25g	30g

1g Fat = 9 calories
1g Carbohydrates = 4 calories
1g Protein = 4 calories

PREPROGRAM NUTRITION LOG

Keep a record of everything you eat for 3 consecutive days. Record all foods and beverages you consume, breaking each food item into its component parts (for example, a turkey sandwich would be listed as 2 slices of bread, 3 oz of turkey, 1 tsp of mayonnaise, and so on). Complete the first two columns of the chart during the course of the day; fill in the remaining information at the end of the day using the Food Guide Pyramid, the table of food groups and recommended servings, information from food labels, and the appendix at the end of this journal listing the nutritional content of many items from fast-food restaurants.

Preprogram Nutrition Log

DAY 1

Food	Portion Size	Food Group	Number of Servings*

*Your portion sizes may be smaller or larger than the serving sizes given in the Food Guide Pyramid; list the actual number of Food Guide Pyramid servings contained in the foods you eat.

Preprogram Nutrition Log

DAY 2

Food	Portion Size	Food Group	Number of Servings*

*Your portion sizes may be smaller or larger than the serving sizes given in the Food Guide Pyramid; list the actual number of Food Guide Pyramid servings contained in the foods you eat.

Preprogram Nutrition Log

DAY 3

Food	Portion Size	Food Group	Number of Servings*

*Your portion sizes may be smaller or larger than the serving sizes given in the Food Guide Pyramid; list the actual number of Food Guide Pyramid servings contained in the foods you eat.

ASSESSING YOUR DAILY DIET

A balanced diet follows the Food Guide Pyramid recommendations. Fill in the actual number of servings from each food group that you recorded, and compare them to the recommended number of servings.

DAY 1 TOTAL

Food Group	Recommended Servings	Actual Servings
Milk, yogurt, cheese	2–3	
Meat, poultry, fish, dry beans, eggs, nuts	2–3	
Fruits	2–4	
Vegetables	3–5	
Breads, cereals, rice, pasta	6–11	
Fats, oils, sweets	use sparingly	

DAY 2 TOTAL

Food Group	Recommended Servings	Actual Servings
Milk, yogurt, cheese	2–3	
Meat, poultry, fish, dry beans, eggs, nuts	2–3	
Fruits	2–4	
Vegetables	3–5	
Breads, cereals, rice, pasta	6–11	
Fats, oils, sweets	use sparingly	

DAY 3 TOTAL

Food Group	Recommended Servings	Actual Servings
Milk, yogurt, cheese	2–3	
Meat, poultry, fish, dry beans, eggs, nuts	2–3	
Fruits	2–4	
Vegetables	3–5	
Breads, cereals, rice, pasta	6–11	
Fats, oils, sweets	use sparingly	

USING A BEHAVIOR CHANGE CONTRACT

Have you identified some areas of your diet where you don't meet the Food Guide Pyramid recommendations? Perhaps you have more than the recommended servings of meat in your diet or fall short in your intake of vegetables. Take a good look at your current diet and think about the changes you can make to improve it. If you need help deciding what kinds of changes you should include in the contract, skip ahead to Tools for Improving Your Food Choices and use the quizzes and tables found there. When you have a good idea of the ways in which you can improve your diet, use the Behavior Change Contract on the next page to record the changes in your diet that you plan to make and the steps that you will follow to reach your goal. (Refer to Chapter 1 in your text for more information on behavior change.)

Behavior Change Contract

1. I ________________________________ agree to

____

2. I will begin on ______________ and plan to reach my goal of ____________________ by ______________

3. In order to reach my final goal, I have devised the following schedule of mini-goals. For each step in my program, I will give myself the reward listed:

Mini-goal	Target date	Reward
____________	________	________
____________	________	________
____________	________	________

My overall reward for reaching my final goal will be

____

4. I have analyzed the internal and external factors leading to my target behavior, and I have identified the following actions I can take to change my behavior:

____

____

5. I will use the following tools to monitor my progress toward reaching my final goal:

____

____

I sign this contract as an indication of my personal commitment to reach my goal.

Your signature: ____________________ Date: __________

I have recruited a helper who will witness my contract and

____

____

Witness signature: ____________________ Date: __________

TOOLS FOR IMPROVING YOUR FOOD CHOICES

Dietary Guidelines for Americans

As you plan to change your diet, keep in mind the Dietary Guidelines for Americans:

- Eat a variety of foods.
- Balance the food you eat with physical activity—maintain or improve your weight.
- Choose a diet with plenty of grain products, vegetables, and fruits.
- Choose a diet low in fat, saturated fat, and cholesterol.
- Choose a diet moderate in sugars.
- Choose a diet moderate in salt and sodium.
- If you drink alcoholic beverages, do so in moderation.

Making Healthy Ethnic Food Choices

	Choose Often	Choose Seldom
Chinese	Chinese Greens Hunan or Szechuan dishes Rice, brown or white Steamed dishes Stir-fry dishes Wonton soup	Crispy duck or beef Egg rolls or fried wontons General Tso's chicken Kung pao dishes Rice, fried Sweet-and-sour dishes
Italian	Cioppino (seafood stew) Minestrone soup, vegetarian Pasta with marinara sauce Pasta primavera Pasta with red or white clam sauce	Cannelloni, ravioli, or manicotti Fettucini alfredo Fried calamari Garlic bread Veal or eggplant parmigiana

	Choose Often	Choose Seldom
Indian	Chapati, (baked tortilla-like bread) Dal (lentils) Karhi (chick-pea soup) Khur (milk and rice dessert) Tandoori, chicken or fish Yogurt-based curry dishes	Bhatura, poori, or paratha (fried breads) Coconut milk–based dishes Ghee (clarified butter) Korma (rich meat dish) Pakoras (fried appetizer) Samosa (fried meat and vegetables in dough)
Japanese	Kushiyaki (broiled foods on skewers) Shabu-shabu (foods in boiling broth) Sushi	Agemono (deep-fried foods) Sukiyaki Tonkatsu (fried pork) Tempura (fried chicken, shrimp, or vegetables)
Mexican	Beans and rice Black bean and vegetable soup Burritos, bean or chicken Fajitas, chicken or vegetable Gazpacho Refried beans, nonfat or low-fat Tortillas, steamed	Chiles rellenos Chimichangas or flautas Enchiladas, beef or cheese Nachos or fried tortillas Quesadillas Refried beans made with lard Taco salad
Thai	Forest salad Larb (chicken salad with mint) Po tak (seafood stew) Yum neua (broiled beef with onions)	Fried fish, duck, or chicken Curries with coconut milk Dishes with peanut sauce Yum koon chaing (sausage with peppers)

Self-Assessment: What Triggers Your Eating?

Hunger isn't the only reason people eat. Efforts to make healthy eating choices can be sabotaged by eating related to other factors, such as emotions or patterns of thinking. Your score on this quiz will help you understand your motiva-tions for eating so that you can create an effective plan for changing your eating behavior. Circle the number that indicates to what degree each situation is likely to make you start eating.

Social	**Very Unlikely**									**Very Likely**
1. Arguing or being in conflict with someone	1	2	3	4	5	6	7	8	9	10
2. Being with others when they are eating	1	2	3	4	5	6	7	8	9	10
3. Being urged to eat by someone else	1	2	3	4	5	6	7	8	9	10
4. Feeling inadequate around others	1	2	3	4	5	6	7	8	9	10
Emotional										
5. Feeling bad, such as being anxious or depressed	1	2	3	4	5	6	7	8	9	10
6. Feeling good, happy, or released	1	2	3	4	5	6	7	8	9	10
7. Feeling bored or having time on my hands	1	2	3	4	5	6	7	8	9	10
8. Feeling stressed or excited	1	2	3	4	5	6	7	8	9	10
Situational										
9. Seeing an advertisement for food or eating	1	2	3	4	5	6	7	8	9	10
10. Passing by a bakery, cookie shop, or other enticement to eat	1	2	3	4	5	6	7	8	9	10
11. Being involved in a party, celebration, or special occasion	1	2	3	4	5	6	7	8	9	10
12. Eating out	1	2	3	4	5	6	7	8	9	10

Thinking	Very Unlikely						Very Likely			
13. Making excuses to myself about why it's okay to eat	1	2	3	4	5	6	7	8	9	10
14. Berating myself for being so fat or unable to control my eating	1	2	3	4	5	6	7	8	9	10
15. Worrying about others or about difficulties I am having	1	2	3	4	5	6	7	8	9	10
16. Thinking about how things should or shouldn't be	1	2	3	4	5	6	7	8	9	10
Physiological										
17. Experiencing pain or discomfort	1	2	3	4	5	6	7	8	9	10
18. Experiencing trembling, headache, or light-headedness associated with no eating or too much caffeine	1	2	3	4	5	6	7	8	9	10
19. Experiencing fatigue or feeling overtired	1	2	3	4	5	6	7	8	9	10
20. Experiencing hunger pangs or urges to eat, even though I've eaten recently	1	2	3	4	5	6	7	8	9	10

Scoring

Total your scores for each area and enter them below. Then rank the scores by marking the highest score "1," next highest score "2," and so on. Focus on the highest-ranked areas first, but any score above 24 is high and indicates that you need to work on that area.

Area	Total Score	Rank Score
Social (Items 1–4)	________	________
Emotional (Items 5–8)	________	________
Situational (Items 9–12)	________	________
Thinking (Items 13–16)	________	________
Physiological (Items 17–20)	________	________

Lowering a High Score

Social Try reducing your susceptibility to the influence of others by communicating more assertively and rethinking your beliefs about obligations you feel you must fulfill.

Emotional Develop stress-management skills and practice positive self-talk to cope with emotions in ways that don't involve food.

Situational Work on controlling your environment and having a plan for handling external cues.

Thinking Change your thinking—be less self-critical and more flexible—to recognize rationalizations and excuses about eating behavior.

Physiological Look at the way you eat, what you eat, and medications to find ways these factors may be affecting your eating behavior.

POSTPROGRAM NUTRITION LOG

Now that you have analyzed your diet and targeted some changes described in your Behavior Change Contract, you are ready to put your plan into action. Fill out this second nutrition log, again keeping a record of everything you eat for 3 consecutive days. Remember to record all foods and beverages you consume, breaking each food item into its component parts (for example, a turkey sandwich would be listed as 2 slices of bread, 3 oz of turkey, 1 tsp of mayon-naise, and so on). Complete the first two columns of the chart during the course of the day; fill in the remaining information at the end of the day using the Food Guide Pyramid, the food groups and recommended servings table, information from food labels, and the appendix listing the nutritional content of many items from fast-food restaurants.

Postprogram Nutrition Log

DAY 1

Food	Portion Size	Food Group	Number of Servings*

*Your portion sizes may be smaller or larger than the serving sizes given in the Food Guide Pyramid; list the actual number of Food Guide Pyramid servings contained in the foods you eat.

Postprogram Nutrition Log

DAY 2

Food	Portion Size	Food Group	Number of Servings*

*Your portion sizes may be smaller or larger than the serving sizes given in the Food Guide Pyramid; list the actual number of Food Guide Pyramid servings contained in the foods you eat.

Postprogram Nutrition Log

DAY 3

Food	Portion Size	Food Group	Number of Servings*

*Your portion sizes may be smaller or larger than the serving sizes given in the Food Guide Pyramid; list the actual number of Food Guide Pyramid servings contained in the foods you eat.

ASSESSING IMPROVEMENT IN YOUR DAILY DIET

Fill in the actual number of servings from each food group that you recorded in your Postprogram Nutrition Log, and compare them to the recommended number of servings. To check your progress, transfer the results from the Preprogram Nutrition Log that you filled out and analyze your new diet for improvement.

DAY 1 TOTAL

Food Group	Recommended Servings	Actual Servings	Preprogram Servings
Milk, yogurt, cheese	2–3		
Meat, poultry, fish, dry beans, eggs, nuts	2–3		
Fruits	2–4		
Vegetables	3–5		
Breads, cereals, rice, pasta	6–11		
Fats, oils, sweets	use sparingly		

DAY 2 TOTAL

Food Group	Recommended Servings	Actual Servings	Preprogram Servings
Milk, yogurt, cheese	2–3		
Meat, poultry, fish, dry beans, eggs, nuts	2–3		
Fruits	2–4		
Vegetables	3–5		
Breads, cereals, rice, pasta	6–11		
Fats, oils, sweets	use sparingly		

DAY 3 TOTAL

Food Group	Recommended Servings	Actual Servings	Preprogram Servings
Milk, yogurt, cheese	2–3		
Meat, poultry, fish, dry beans, eggs, nuts	2–3		
Fruits	2–4		
Vegetables	3–5		
Breads, cereals, rice, pasta	6–11		
Fats, oils, sweets	use sparingly		

In comparing the results of my Postprogram Nutrition Log to the results of my preprogram log, I found that

____

____

Completing a Behavior Change Contract and following its steps helped me to

____

____

____

Areas of improvement that I will focus on in the future are

____

____

____

____

____

____

____

WEIGHT MANAGEMENT

CREATING A WEIGHT MANAGEMENT PROGRAM

Completing the preprogram and postprogram nutrition logs will help you monitor and improve your daily diet. If you decide that your weight is above or below the amount that is appropriate for your size, gender, and age, the information you have gathered with your nutrition logs will be an important part of a weight management program. This section outlines the general steps in a weight management program; in the next section you'll track activity and food choices to identify ways to create a negative energy balance and lose weight.

Follow these steps to develop your weight management program and put it into action:

1. Assess Your Motivation and Commitment
Make sure you are motivated and committed to your plan for weight management before you begin. It is important to understand why you want to change your weight. You will generally be more successful if your reasons are self-focused, such as wanting to feel good about yourself, rather than connected to others' perceptions of you.

When you understand your reasons for wanting to manage your weight, list them below. Post your list in a prominent place as a reminder.

1. ______________________________

2. ______________________________

3. ______________________________

4. ______________________________

2. Set Goals

After you have chosen a reasonable long-term weight or body-fat percentage goal, break your progress into a series of short-term goals. You can include a small, non-food-related reward like a new CD or a night at the movies for successfully reaching each goal.

	Goal	Reward
1.	____________________	________________________
2.	____________________	________________________
3.	____________________	________________________
4.	____________________	________________________

3. Assess Your Current Energy Balance

When your weight is stable, you are burning approximately the same number of calories that you are taking in. In order to lose weight, you must consume fewer calories, burn more calories through physical activity, or both. This will create a negative energy balance that will lead to gradual, moderate weight loss. Strategies for creating a negative energy balance are discussed on page 29 of this journal.

4. Increase Your Level of Physical Activity

You can increase your energy output simply by increasing your routine physical activity, such as walking or taking the stairs. You will also increase your energy output by adopting a program of regular exercise.

5. Evaluate Your Diet and Eating Habits

Take another look at the nutrition logs you completed. Are there some high-calorie or high-fat foods that stand out? If your increase in physical activity does not result in a negative energy balance that produces weight loss, you may want to make small cuts in your calorie intake by reducing your consumption of these foods.

6. Track Your Physical Activity and Diet
Use the weight management logs to record your physical activities and dietary choices. These logs will help you uncover potential calorie savings that will create a negative calorie balance and help you lose weight.

For People Who Want to Gain Weight

If the goal of your weight management program is to increase your weight, you'll need to create a positive energy balance by taking in more calories than you use. The basis of a successful and healthy program for weight gain is a combination of strength training and a high-calorie diet. Strength training will help you add weight as muscle rather than as fat. To increase your calorie consumption, eat more high-carbohydrate foods, including grains, vegetables, and fruits. (Fatty, high-calorie foods may seem like a logical choice for weight gain, but a diet high in fat carries health risks, and your body is likely to convert dietary fat into body fat rather than into muscle.) Avoid skipping meals, add two or three snacks to your daily diet, and consider adding a dietary supplement high in carbohydrates, protein, vitamins, and minerals. As with weight loss, a gradual program of weight gain is the best strategy.

CREATING A NEGATIVE ENERGY BALANCE

A reasonable weight-loss goal is 1/2–1 pound per week. Depending on your individual characteristics, you will need to create a negative energy balance of between 1750 and 3500 calories a week, or 250–500 calories a day. While this may seem daunting, you already make choices every day that affect your energy balance significantly. Making a few decisions each day with your energy balance in mind can add up to a successful weight management program.

First, review the sample weight management log on the next page that shows the daily activities of Elizabeth, a hypothetical 21-year-old student weighing 130 pounds. As she goes through her day, she has many opportunities to make choices that will affect her energy balance. In the real world, you will be more likely to make one or two choices each day that decrease the number of calories you take in or increase the number of calories you expend. The key is to be aware of your opportunities to affect your energy balance and to make healthy choices as often as possible without making yourself feel deprived.

After you have reviewed this example, record and assess your own daily choices using the blank weight management logs that follow. Fill in your activities and your meals and snacks, and then think about alternatives you could have chosen. What would the potential calorie savings have been if you had made these choices? To calculate the calories you expended in physical activity, consult the table of common sports and fitness activities on page 33 of this journal and, from your textbook, examples of moderate physical activity (Figure 2-1) on page 22 and the more complete summary of sports and fitness activities (Table 7-1) on page 160. To calculate calories saved by making a healthier food choice, use Appendix B, Nutritional Content of Common Foods. Another of your textbook's appendixes, Nutritional Content of Popular Items from Fast-Food Restaurants, can also be found at the back of this journal for quick reference.

Sample Daily Weight Management Log

Activity/Meal or Snack	Healthier Choice (describe)	Approximate Calorie Savings
Friday morning, Elizabeth eats breakfast: a croissant and a cup of coffee with cream.	Friday morning, Elizabeth eats breakfast: a bowl of whole-grain cereal, a glass of orange juice, and a cup of coffee. She uses most of a glass of skim milk for her cereal and puts the rest in her coffee.	81
Elizabeth drives to campus.	Elizabeth walks 15 minutes to campus.	57
After class, Elizabeth visits her friend's dorm, where they watch the noon soap opera for an hour.	After class, Elizabeth meets her friend for a 25-minute jog.	195
For lunch, Elizabeth eats 2 slices of leftover pepperoni pizza and drinks a soda.	After their jog, they have lunch at the dorm; each has a turkey sandwich, an apple, and iced tea.	231
Elizabeth goes to her afternoon class. She wants a snack, so she buys a candy bar from the vending machine.	Elizabeth goes to her afternoon class. She wants a snack, so she buys a nonfat yogurt with fruit in the student union.	142
Elizabeth drives home.	Elizabeth walks 15 minutes home.	57
Elizabeth studies until her roommates get home.	Elizabeth studies until her roommates get home.	—
Elizabeth and her roommates decide to stop for fast food on the way to the movies. Elizabeth orders a cheeseburger, large french fries, and a small chocolate shake.	Elizabeth and her roommates decide to stop for fast food on the way to the movies. Elizabeth orders a hamburger, a green salad with carrots and fat-free dressing, and a small chocolate shake.	389
At the movies, Elizabeth shares a bag of buttered popcorn with her friend.	At the movies, Elizabeth shares a bag of air-popped popcorn with her friend.	64

Daily Weight Management Log

Activity/Meal or Snack	Healthier Choice (describe)	Approximate Calorie Savings

Daily Weight Management Log

Activity/Meal or Snack	Healthier Choice (describe)	Approximate Calorie Savings

COMMON SPORTS AND FITNESS ACTIVITIES

When you change your energy balance by participating in an activity that expends calories, how do you calculate how many calories you have actually spent? Calorie costs are given here for 10 common activities. If you have chosen an activity not listed here, consult Table 7-1, A Summary of Sports and Fitness Activities, on page 160 of your textbook.

Multiply the number in the appropriate column (moderate or vigorous) by your body weight and then by the number of minutes you exercise. (If you participate in your activity at a level between moderate and vigorous, use a number between the two values.) For example, if you weigh 150 pounds and play tennis vigorously for 45 minutes, you multiply .071 (value) by 150 (weight) and then by 45 (time) for a result of 479 calories expended.

	Approximate Calorie Cost	
Activity	*Moderate*	*Vigorous*
Aerobic dance	.046	.062
Basketball, half court	.045	.071
Bicycling	.049	.071
Hiking	.051	.073
Jogging and running	.060	.104
Racquetball, skilled, singles	.049	.078
Skating, ice, roller, and in-line	.045	.095
Swimming	.032	.088
Tennis, skilled, singles	—	.071
Walking	.029	.048

Nutritional Content of Popular Items from Fast Food Restaurants

Arby's

	Serving size	Calories	Protein	Total fat	Saturated fat	Total carbohydrate	Sugars	Fiber	Cholesterol	Sodium	Vitamin A	Vitamin C	Calcium	Iron	% calories from fat
	g		g	g	g	g	g	g	mg	mg	% Daily Value				
Regular roast beef	154	388	23	19	7	33	N/A	3	43	1009	N/A	N/A	N/A	N/A	44
Super roast beef	247	523	25	27	9	50	N/A	5	43	1189	N/A	N/A	N/A	N/A	46
Light roast beef deluxe	182	296	18	10	3	33	N/A	6	42	826	N/A	N/A	N/A	N/A	30
Roast chicken deluxe	216	433	24	22	5	36	N/A	2	34	763	N/A	N/A	N/A	N/A	46
French dip	195	475	30	22	8	40	N/A	3	55	1411	N/A	N/A	N/A	N/A	41
Turkey sub	277	550	31	27	7	47	N/A	2	65	2084	N/A	N/A	N/A	N/A	44
Light roast turkey deluxe	195	260	20	7	2	33	N/A	4	33	1262	N/A	N/A	N/A	N/A	21
Grilled chicken BBQ	201	388	23	13	3	47	N/A	2	43	1002	N/A	N/A	N/A	N/A	30
Cheddar curly fries	120	333	5	18	4	40	N/A	0	3	1016	N/A	N/A	N/A	N/A	49
Potato cakes	85	204	2	12	2	20	N/A	0	0	397	N/A	N/A	N/A	N/A	53
Red ranch dressing	14	75	0	6	1	5	N/A	0	0	115	N/A	N/A	N/A	N/A	72
French-toastix	124	430	10	21	5	52	N/A	3	0	550	N/A	N/A	N/A	N/A	44
Jamocha shake	340	384	15	10	3	62	N/A	0	36	262	N/A	N/A	N/A	N/A	23

N/A: not available.

Burger King

	Serving size	Calories	Protein	Total fat	Saturated fat	Total carbohydrate	Sugars	Fiber	Cholesterol	Sodium	Vitamin A	Vitamin C	Calcium	Iron	% calories from fat
	g		g	g	g	g	g	g	mg	mg	% Daily Value				
Whopper®	270	640	27	39	11	45	8	3	90	870	N/A	N/A	N/A	N/A	55
Whopper Jr.®	164	420	21	24	8	29	5	2	60	530	N/A	N/A	N/A	N/A	51
Double Whopper® with cheese	375	960	52	63	24	46	8	3	195	1420	N/A	N/A	N/A	N/A	59
BK Big Fish™ sandwich	252	720	23	43	9	59	4	3	80	1180	N/A	N/A	N/A	N/A	54
BK Broiler® chicken sandwich	247	530	29	26	5	5	4	2	105	1060	N/A	N/A	N/A	N/A	44
Chicken Tenders® (8 pieces)	123	350	22	22	7	17	0	1	65	940	N/A	N/A	N/A	N/A	57
Ranch dipping sauce	28	170	0	17	3	2	1	0	0	200	N/A	N/A	N/A	N/A	90
Barbeque dipping sauce	28	35	0	0	0	9	7	0	0	400	N/A	N/A	N/A	N/A	0
Broiled chicken salad (no dressing)	302	190	20	8	4	9	5	3	75	500	N/A	N/A	N/A	N/A	38
Garden salad (no dressing)	215	100	6	5	3	8	4	4	15	115	N/A	N/A	N/A	N/A	45
Bleu cheese salad dressing	30	160	2	16	4	1	0	<1	30	260	N/A	N/A	N/A	N/A	90
French fries (medium, salted)	116	400	3	21	8	50	0	4	0	820	N/A	N/A	N/A	N/A	47
Onion rings	124	310	4	14	2	41	6	6	0	810	N/A	N/A	N/A	N/A	41
Chocolate shake (medium)	284	320	9	7	4	54	48	3	20	230	N/A	N/A	N/A	N/A	20
Croissan'wich® w/sausage, egg, and cheese	176	600	22	46	16	25	3	1	260	1140	N/A	N/A	N/A	N/A	69
French toast sticks	141	500	4	27	7	60	11	1	0	490	N/A	N/A	N/A	N/A	49
Dutch apple pie	113	300	3	15	3	39	22	2	0	230	N/A	N/A	N/A	N/A	45

N/A: not available.

Domino's Pizza

(1 serving = 2 of 12 slices or ⅙ of 14-inch pizza; 2 of 8 slices or ¼ of 12-inch pizza; 1 6-inch pizza)

	Serving size	Calories	Protein	Total fat	Saturated fat	Total carbohydrate	Sugars	Fiber	Cholesterol	Sodium	Vitamin A	Vitamin C	Calcium	Iron	% calories from fat
	g		g	g	g	g	g	g	mg	mg	% Daily Value				
14-inch lg. hand-tossed cheese	137	317	13	10	5	45	3	3	14	669	10	9	17	18	28
14-inch lg. thin crust cheese	99	253	11	11	5	29	2	2	14	757	9	4	20	5	39
14-inch lg. deep dish cheese	173	455	18	20	8	54	5	3	18	1029	11	5	22	21	39
12-inch med. hand-tossed cheese	149	347	14	11	5	50	3	3	15	723	11	8	18	20	29
12-inch med. thin crust cheese	106	271	12	12	5	31	3	2	15	509	10	4	22	5	40
12-inch med. deep dish cheese	180	477	18	22	8	55	5	3	19	1085	12	5	23	21	42
6-inch deep dish cheese	215	595	23	27	11	68	6	4	24	1300	13	5	28	26	41
Toppings: pepperoni	*	66	3	6	2	<1	<1	<1	14	212	†	†	†	†	82
ham	*	17	2	1	<1	<1	<1	0	7	156	†	†	†	†	53
Italian sausage	*	44	2	3	1	1	<1	<1	9	137	†	†	†	†	61
bacon	*	75	4	6	2	<1	<1	0	11	207	†	7	†	†	72
beef	*	44	2	4	2	<1	<1	<1	8	123	†	†	†	†	82
anchovies	*	23	3	1	<1	0	0	0	9	395	†	†	3	3	39
extra cheese	*	45	3	4	2	<1	<1	<1	7	140	3	†	12	†	80
cheddar cheese	*	48	3	4	2	<1	<1	0	12	73	3	†	9	†	75
Barbeque wings	25	50	6	2	1	2	1	<1	26	175	†	†	†	†	38
Hot wings	25	45	6	2	1	<1	<1	<1	26	354	3	†	†	†	40
Breadsticks (1 piece)	22	78	2	3	1	11	<1	<1	0	158	†	†	†	3	35
Cheesy bread (1 piece)	28	103	3	5	2	11	<1	<1	6	187	†	26	†	4	44

* Topping information is based on minimal portioning requirements for one serving of a 14-inch large pizza; add the values for toppings to the values for a cheese pizza. The following toppings supply fewer than 15 calories per serving: green and yellow peppers, onion, olives, mushrooms, pineapple.

† Contains less than 2% of the Daily Value of these nutrients.

Jack in the Box

	Serving size	Calories	Protein	Total fat	Saturated fat	Total carbohydrate	Sugars	Fiber	Cholesterol	Sodium	Vitamin A	Vitamin C	Calcium	Iron	% calories from fat
	g		g	g	g	g	g	g	mg	mg	% Daily Value				
Breakfast Jack®	126	280	17	12	5	30	3	1	195	920	8	4	15	20	39
Supreme croissant	163	520	21	32	13	39	6	2	245	1240	15	20	10	20	57
Hamburger	97	280	13	11	4	31	5	1	45	560	2	2	10	20	39
Jumbo Jack®	263	590	25	36	11	42	6	4	80	720	8	20	15	35	55
Sourdough Jack	229	690	31	46	15	38	3	3	110	1180	10	15	30	20	60
Chicken fajita pita	187	280	24	9	4	25	5	3	75	840	25	0	15	15	29
Grilled chicken fillet	231	520	27	26	6	42	9	4	140	1240	8	15	20	25	45
Chicken supreme	235	680	23	45	11	46	8	4	85	1500	10	15	20	15	60
Chicken Caesar sandwich	232	490	24	26	6	41	6	3	55	1050	15	15	20	20	48
Garden chicken salad	253	200	23	9	4	8	4	3	65	420	70	20	20	4	41
Blue cheese dressing	57	210	1	15	2.5	11	4	0	25	750	0	0	2	0	64
Chicken teriyaki bowl	502	670	26	4	1	128	27	3	15	1730	130	40	10	25	5
Monster taco	125	270	12	17	6	19	2	4	30	678	8	2	20	8	57
Egg rolls (3 pieces)	170	440	15	24	6	40	5	4	35	1020	15	20	8	25	49
Chicken breast pieces (5)	150	360	27	17	3	24	0	1	80	970	4	2	2	10	39
Stuffed jalapeños (10 pieces)	240	750	20	44	17	65	7	5	80	2470	30	50	45	10	53
Barbeque dipping sauce	28	45	1	0	0	11	7	0	0	310	0	0	0	0	0
Seasoned curly fries	125	410	6	23	5	45	0	4	0	1010	6	0	4	10	50
Onion rings	120	460	7	25	5	50	3	3	0	780	4	30	4	15	49
Cappuccino ice cream shake	16*	630	11	29	17	80	58	0	90	320	15	0	35	0	41

*Fluid ounces

KFC

	Serving size	Calories	Protein	Total fat	Saturated fat	Total carbohydrate	Sugars	Fiber	Cholesterol	Sodium	Vitamin A	Vitamin C	Calcium	Iron	% calories from fat
	g		g	g	g	g	g	g	mg	mg	% Daily Value				
Original Recipe®: breast	153	400	29	24	6	16	0	1	135	1116	*	*	4	6	54
thigh	91	250	16	18	4.5	6	0	1	95	747	*	*	2	4	65
Extra Tasty Crispy™: breast	168	470	31	28	7	25	0	1	80	930	*	*	4	6	54
thigh	118	370	19	25	6	18	0	2	70	540	*	*	2	4	61
Hot & Spicy: breast	180	530	32	35	8	23	0	2	110	1110	*	*	4	6	59
thigh	107	370	18	27	7	13	0	1	90	570	*	*	*	4	66
Tender Roast™: breast (as served)	139	251	37	11	3	1	<1	0	151	830	*	*	*	*	39
breast (skin removed)	118	169	31	4	1	1	0	0	112	797	*	*	*	*	21
thigh (as served)	90	207	18	12	4	<2	<1	0	120	504	*	*	*	*	52
thigh (skin removed)	59	106	13	6	2	<1	<1	0	84	312	*	*	*	*	51
Hot Wings™ Pieces	135	471	27	33	8	18	0	2	150	1230	*	*	4	8	63
Colonel's Crispy Strips™ (3)	92	261	20	16	4	10	0	3	40	658	*	*	*	3	55
Chunky chicken pot pie	368	770	29	42	13	69	8	5	70	2160	80	2	10	10	49
Corn on the cob	162	150	5	2	0	35	8	2	0	20	2	6	*	*	12
Mashed potatoes w/gravy	136	120	1	6	1	17	0	2	<1	440	*	*	*	2	45
Mean Greens™	152	70	4	3	1	11	1	5	10	650	60	10	20	10	39
BBQ baked beans	156	190	6	3	1	33	13	6	5	760	8	*	8	10	14
Potato salad	160	230	4	14	2	23	9	23	15	540	10	*	2	15	55
Cole slaw	142	180	2	9	1.5	21	20	3	5	280	*	60	4	4	45
Biscuit (1)	56	180	4	10	2.5	20	2	<1	0	560	*	*	2	6	50

*Contains less than 2% of the Daily Value of these nutrients.

McDonald's

	Serving size	Calories	Protein	Total fat	Saturated fat	Total carbohydrate	Sugars	Fiber	Cholesterol	Sodium	Vitamin A	Vitamin C	Calcium	Iron	% calories from fat
	g		g	g	g	g	g	g	mg	mg	% Daily Value				
Hamburger	107	260	13	9	3.5	34	7	2	30	580	*	4	15	15	31
Cheeseburger	121	320	15	13	6	35	7	2	40	820	6	4	20	15	37
Quarter-Pounder®	172	420	23	21	8	37	8	2	70	820	2	4	30	25	45
Quarter-Pounder® w/cheese	200	530	28	30	13	38	9	2	95	1290	10	4	15	25	51
Big Mac®	216	560	26	31	10	45	8	3	85	1070	6	4	25	25	50
Arch Deluxe™	239	550	29	31	11	39	8	4	90	1010	10	10	15	25	51
Fish Filet Deluxe™	228	560	23	28	6	54	5	4	60	1060	6	4	8	15	45
Grilled Chicken Deluxe™	223	440	27	20	3	38	6	4	60	1040	6	8	6	15	41
French fries (large)	147	450	6	22	4	57	0	5	0	290	*	30	2	6	44
Chicken McNuggets® (6 pieces)	106	290	18	17	3.5	15	0	0	60	510	*	*	2	6	53
Barbeque sauce	28	45	0	0	0	10	10	0	0	250	*	6	*	*	0
Garden salad (no dressing)	177	35	2	0	0	7	3	3	0	20	120	40	4	6	0
Grilled chicken salad (no dressing)	257	120	21	1.5	0	7	3	3	45	240	120	25	4	8	1
Ranch dressing (1 pkg.)	N/A	230	1	21	3	10	6	0	20	550	*	2	4	*	82
Fat-free herb vinaigrette (1 pkg.)	N/A	50	0	0	0	11	9	0	0	330	*	2	*	2	0
Egg McMuffin®	136	290	17	12	4.5	27	3	1	235	790	10	2	20	15	37
Hash browns	53	130	1	8	1.5	14	0	1	0	330	*	4	*	2	55
Hotcakes w/margarine & syrup	222	570	9	16	3	100	42	2	15	750	8	*	10	15	25
Chocolate shake, small	N/A	360	11	9	6	60	54	1	40	250	6	2	35	4	23
Baked apple pie	77	260	3	13	3.5	34	13	<1	0	200	*	40	2	6	45

*Contains less than 2% of the Daily Value of these nutrients.

Taco Bell

	Serving size	Calories	Protein	Total fat	Saturated fat	Total carbohydrate	Sugars	Fiber	Cholesterol	Sodium	Vitamin A	Vitamin C	Calcium	Iron	% calories from fat
	oz		g	g	g	g	g	g	mg	mg	% Daily Value				
Taco	2.75	180	9	10	4	12	1	3	25	330	10	0	8	6	50
Taco Supreme®	4	220	10	14	6	14	2	3	35	350	15	6	10	6	57
Double Decker Taco Supreme®	7	390	15	19	8	40	3	9	35	760	15	6	15	10	44
BLT soft taco	4.5	340	11	23	8	22	3	2	40	610	4	6	10	4	61
Burrito Supreme®	9	440	17	19	8	51	4	10	35	1230	50	8	15	15	39
Big Beef Burrito Supreme®	10.5	520	17	23	10	54	4	11	55	1520	60	8	15	15	40
Chili cheese burrito	5	330	10	13	6	37	2	5	35	870	60	0	20	8	35
Beef Gorditas Supreme®	5	300	21	13	6	31	3	3	35	390	10	4	8	15	39
Chicken Gorditas Supreme®	5	290	14	12	5	30	4	2	55	420	10	4	8	10	37
Big Beef MexiMelt®	4.75	290	21	15	7	23	0	4	45	850	25	6	20	6	47
Taco salad	19	850	9	52	15	65	1	16	60	1780	160	40	30	35	55
Taco salad w/o shell	16.5	420	5	21	11	32	1	15	60	1520	160	35	25	25	47
Chicken Fajita Wrap™	8	470	9	21	6	51		4	60	1290	35	6	15	8	42
Veggie Fajita Wrap™	8	420		19	5	53		3	20	980	35	6	15	8	41
Steak Fajita Wrap™ Supreme	9	510		25	8	52		3	50	1200	30	10	15	10	44
Big Beef Nachos Supreme	7	450		24	8	45		9	30	810	10	6	15	15	48
Nachos BellGrande®	11	720		39	11	84		17	35	1310	15	6	20	20	46
Pintos 'n cheese	4.5	190		9	4	18		10	15	650	50	0	15	10	43
Mexican rice	4.75	190		9	3.5	23		1	15	760	100	2	15	8	43
Fiesta breakfast burrito	3.5	280		16	6	25		2	25	580	15	0	8	4	51

Wendy's

	Serving size	Calories	Protein	Total fat	Saturated fat	Total carbohydrate	Sugars	Fiber	Cholesterol	Sodium	Vitamin A	Vitamin C	Calcium	Iron	% calories from fat
	g		g	g	g	g	g	g	mg	mg	% Daily Value				
Single w/everything	219	420	25	20	7	37	9	3	70	920	6	10	13	26	43
Big Bacon Classic	282	580	34	30	12	46	11	3	100	1460	15	25	25	30	47
Jr. hamburger	118	270	15	10	3.5	34	7	2	30	610	2	2	11	17	33
Jr. bacon cheeseburger	166	380	20	19	7	34	7	2	60	850	8	10	17	19	45
Grilled chicken sandwich	189	310	27	8	1.5	35	8	2	65	790	4	10	10	15	23
Caesar side salad (no dressing)	92	110	10	5	2.5	7	1	1	15	650	35	25	15	6	41
Grilled chicken salad (no dressing)	338	200	25	8	1.5	9	6	3	50	720	120	60	19	11	36
Taco salad (no dressing)	468	380	26	19	10	28	9	7	65	1040	45	45	37	23	45
Blue cheese dressing (2T)	28	180	1	19	3	0	0	0	15	180	2	0	2	0	95
Ranch dressing, reduced fat (2T)	28	60	1	5	1	2	1	0	10	240	0	0	1	0	75
Soft breadstick	44	130	4	3	0.5	23	N/A	1	5	250	0	0	4	9	21
French fries, medium	130	390	5	19	3	50	0	5	0	120	0	10	2	6	44
Baked potato w/broccoli & cheese	411	470	9	14	2.5	80	6	9	5	470	35	120	21	25	27
Baked potato w/chili & cheese	439	630	20	24	9	83	7	9	40	770	20	60	35	28	34
Chili, small, plain	227	210	15	7	2.5	21	5	5	30	800	8	6	8	16	30
Chili, large w/cheese & crackers	363	405	28	16.5	7	37	8	7	60	1380	14	10	25	26	37
Chicken nuggets (5)	75	230	11	16	3	11	0	0	30	470	0	2	2	2	63
Barbeque sauce	28	45	1	0	0	10	7	0	0	160	0	0	1	3	0
Frosty dairy dessert, medium	298	440	11	11	7	73	56	0	50	260	20	0	41	8	23
Chicken club sandwich	216	470	31	20	4	44	6	2	70	970	4	10	11	17	38

N/A: not available.

Credits

Source for Food Guide Pyramid: U.S. Department of Agriculture, Human Nutrition Information Service. 1996. *Food Guide Pyramid.* Home and Garden Bulletin No. 252.

Source for Self-Assessment: Portion Size Quiz: From What's in a portion? *Tufts University Diet and Nutrition Letter,* September 1994. Used with permission of the publisher.

Source for Self-Assessment: What Triggers Your Eating? Adapted from Nash, J. D. 1997. *The New Maximize Your Body Potential.* Palo Alto, Calif.: Bull Publishing. Reprinted with permission from Bull Publishing Company.

Sources for Making Healthy Ethnic Food Choices: The sat fat switch. 1997. *Nutrition Action Healthletter,* January/ February. University of Southern Florida Student Health Service. 1997. Ethnic food (http://www.shs.usf.edu/Health/ ethnic.html). The best of Asian cuisines. 1993. *University of California at Berkeley Wellness Letter,* January. Eating in ethnic restaurants. 1990. *Runner's World,* January.